NEUROPRESSURE

Unlock your brain's potential

David Corby

Special Note: The described techniques and procedures offered herein, are solely for information and research purposes. The author does not present any part of this work, directly or indirectly, as diagnosis or prescription for any ailment of any reader or trainee. Nor do we recommend these procedures per se, nor make any representation concerning the physiological effects of any of the ideas we report. People who use the techniques in this book do so at their own risk.

Photos: courtesy of David Star, www.soulconnection.net.au

Corby, David, 1969-.
Neuropressure.

ISBN: 978 1 291 57390 9.

More information:
www.davidcorby.net or www.complementary.com.au

TABLE OF CONTENTS

Authors Note

I would like to thank my wife, who through her illness and subsequent recovery established my link with complementary medicine. She is a tremendous support and a wonderful life companion.

Many people have contributed to the development of this book. Above all I would like to thank Alfred Schatz for encouraging me to write this book and providing guidance along the way.

I would like to acknowledge all of my clients, who over the years have been my most important teachers - particularly the more difficult cases who contributed greatly to my understanding and challenged me to learn more about the nature of the mind and body.

This book is based on Vibrational Healing Systems courses I have written and taught to hundreds of students in Australia and overseas, particularly Brain Function 1 which integrates Western approaches to assessing and improving brain function with the Traditional Chinese approach.

I would like to acknowledge the indirect contribution of George Goodheart and Charles Krebs to this work. My exposure to the use of acupoints for improving brain function began in my first kinesiology class where a simplified version of the George Goodheart inspired Applied Kinesiology approach to brain confusion was taught.

While my courses, clinic work and this book's approach to brain function moves away from this concept of brain confusion, it is still built around the idea that acupuncture points can be used to improve brain function. It is true that the Chinese first thought of the idea, but I would not have heard of it if I had not been taught it in kinesiology.

Charles Krebs went much further in his LEAP program. It was in working with LEAP that I received much of the inspiration for this work.

I started working more closely with the Traditional Chinese Medicine approach to brain function when working on a client with Asperger's syndrome. The main impetus at the time was to be able to clear stress in different brain areas more deeply and thoroughly, because it was really needed for this client.

I thought this was achievable if I could find points that are more directly linked to the brain than those that I had been using. I was particularly looking for points that had a long tradition of successful application by the Chinese, and had a wider context that took account of the brain-mind-spirit model.

The results generated by this approach convinced me that I was on the right track, to the point where my work on all learning difficulties clients was based on this system.

I would also like to thank Christopher Rowe and Ondrej Bursik for their support and good ideas.

INTRODUCTION

Welcome to Brain Power. This book has the potential to improve how well you think, memorise, read, move and do just about any type of brain function.

The work that underpins this book changed my life forever.

A few years ago my wife had a severe and potentially life threatening illness (viral encephalitis) that left her unable to speak or hear well. After 9 months she seemed to be getting worse.

We were desperate.

It was just about this time I read a book about kinesiology. We thought it was worth trying so we booked into see a Holistic Kinesiologist.

In the first session she was asked what was her favourite flower and she replied "yellow". She had been thinking of a "white daisy". This was often the best she was able to articulate.

Within five one-hour sessions Anita was significantly better. The fits had stopped and she could speak more fluently. Today she has fully recovered. For us it was a miracle. It gave us our life back.

After this experience I became so interested in Holistic Kinesiology that I changed from working in the financial markets as a Chief Economist to working as a Holistic Kinesiologist.

It is an amazingly effective modality.

While this book does not cover the main information gathering tool of kinesiology – muscle monitoring – we do make use of many of the techniques that helped my wife. In particular we use acupressure to help diffuse stress in the brain and allow the brain to function better.

The techniques are simple and easy to use and often produce profound results quickly.

YOU ARE CAPABLE OF MORE

Most people do not realise how much they are capable of. Many things hold us back from reaching our full brain function potential.

Intelligence and brain function are two different things. Intelligence provides a measure of potential. Brain function relates to what we can actually do. Often people with profound learning difficulties are very intelligent. Their problem is that they cannot make effective use of this intelligence.

What gets in the way of making full use of your intelligence? The answer is stress.

For example, if someone that you have not seen for 20 years comes up and says "Hi" and remembers your name, you will feel pressured to instantly remember their name. The more pressured you feel the less likely you are to remember. Yet the minute they leave and the pressure to remember is removed you suddenly remember their name. Most of us have had moments like this.

Another example is when you sit in an exam trying to remember something that you have learnt. The more stress you feel the less you are able to recall. After the exam is over and the pressure is removed you may suddenly remember the answers.

Our brain can cope only with a certain degree of stress. Function declines once we pass this threshold level of stress. All people lose function as stress increases, although people differ in the amount of stress they can cope with before noticeably losing function.

For some people normal life is sufficiently stressful to impede their brain function. For others particular situations, like speaking in front of three hundred people, or coping with difficult issues at particular times of their life, or a deterioration of health will prompt a loss of brain function.

In this book we will use the acupressure system to alleviate stress – increasing the level of stress you can cope with before losing brain function. We do that by activating an activity that is stressful and then holding an acupressure point to decrease the stress associated with that activity.

The Chinese have used acupressure to improve brain function for thousands of years. I am still astounded by the degree of improvement you can get by holding acupressure points, having seen amazing improvements in a wide variety of common brain function difficulties.

THE IMPORTANCE OF MOVEMENT

Movement is integral for learning.

If you sit and watch babies learn about their environment, you will quickly notice movement and touch form part of nearly every aspect of their learning. Babies try to touch everything, and if possible put everything in their mouth to really activate their touch senses. How often have you heard parents of young children say in shops – "do not touch that." Kids want to touch in order to better understand.

Coordinated movement improves communication between different areas of the brain.

People that move well think well. People that think well also move well. Movement and brain function go hand in hand.

Some therapies use movement to improve brain function. Other therapies target improved brain function in order to improve movement. In my clinic I do both.

A person's level of coordination can be used as a barometer of their level of brain function. Using coordinated movement can also help in improving brain function. Coordinated movement has been used to great effect on even severe brain dysfunctions such as autism.

WHY USE ACUPRESSURE?

The Chinese have been using acupoints to improve brain function for thousands of years. The acupuncture system is closely intertwined with the nervous system. I have found acupressure to produce the quickest results and often be the most effective of all the therapies I have tried.

Holding acupoints can make a major difference to brain function. You can reduce the stress associated with a function by holding a point while doing that function. Holding points directly reduces stress. Different points can be used to target different types of functions and different parts of the brain.

Some points are good for improving coordination while others are good for hearing, sight, concrete thinking and so on.

Recent clinical studies using brain scan (MRI) technology have proven that many of the commonly used points stimulate the very areas of the brain that the Chinese have used them for throughout the last 3000 years of clinical application.

OUR TWO PART PROCESS

The process we use in this book is to :

- ▶ Activate a function that is stressful, such as coordinated movement or reading;
- ▶ Then hold an acupoint that helps reduce the stress associated with this function.

In this book we make use of some of the key acupoints for particular functions. When you hold these acupoints it is best to stay clear and focussed on the points. Wait for the person to calm. If you are holding your own acupoints, find a comfortable position and wait till you feel calm and at peace. A good sign that you have held the points for long enough is when the person's breathing becomes calm and regular.

Often function improves instantly. This happens when the brain has already developed the capacity for doing the function but a stress was making it difficult to do. This is the most common situation.

However, sometimes it can take a while for the function to improve. This happens when a stress or stressors prevented the brain from developing the capacity to do that function well. When we reduce the stress, the brain must then learn to do the function well, laying down new pathways that enable the function to be done efficiently. That takes time (usually a few weeks at least - in many cases several months).

STEP 1

ASSESSING OVERALL BRAIN FUNCTION

You will begin by assessing your level of function. You will do a number of tasks that activate the brain and score each of them. This will serve as a basis for step 2 and for later re-assessment. You can either assess yourself or have someone assess you. If you are assessing yourself you will need to find a large mirror to stand in front of.

You will begin with movement because movement tells us a great deal about the general level of brain function. You should particularly take note of the level of coordination between the arms and legs, because this provides an insight into how well different areas of the brain are able to coordinate – particularly the links between the left and right hemispheres of the brain.

When you march normally, ie moving your right arm and left leg or left arm and right leg, you use both hemispheres of the brain. Your left arm and leg is coordinated by the right hemisphere of the brain. The right arm and leg is coordinated by the left hemisphere of the brain. If you move your left arm and your right leg you must simultaneously use both left and right hemispheres of the brain.

The degree of coordination between the left arm and the right leg gives us an indication of the ease of communication and coordination between the left and right hemispheres of the brain.

SAME SIDE MARCHING

Same side marching is where you use an arm and leg on the same side of the body. Adults do not tend to move this way often. Generally when we walk we move the opposite arm and leg forward. Our nervous system is designed to make this the normal walking movement.

Same sided movements are more common in infants and children. Same sided movements are generally a simpler level of coordination that is used particularly early on in a child's development. For example, if a baby's head turns left, its arm will reach out to the left as well (this is related to some early 'primitive' reflexes that are important in early brain and coordination development). As adults we still use same sided movements at times, although walking and running is generally opposite sided.

Same sided marching is useful for your assessment because it provides an indication of your stress during early brain development. Early brain development is important because it provides the foundation upon which later functions are built. Complex brain functions need to be built on solid foundations, just like the walls of a building are only stable if the foundations are stable.

Adults should be able to do same sided marching without stress. However, I have found many adults struggle with same sided marching even when opposite side marching is reasonably coordinated. When their same sided marching improves many other functions tend to improve and often opposite side marching improves as well.

Assessment 1:

March on the spot moving the arm and leg of one side of the body followed by the arm and leg of the other side of the body (see picture below). For example move the left arm and leg, then the right arm and leg and so on.

Picture heading: **Same Side Marching**

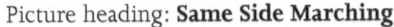

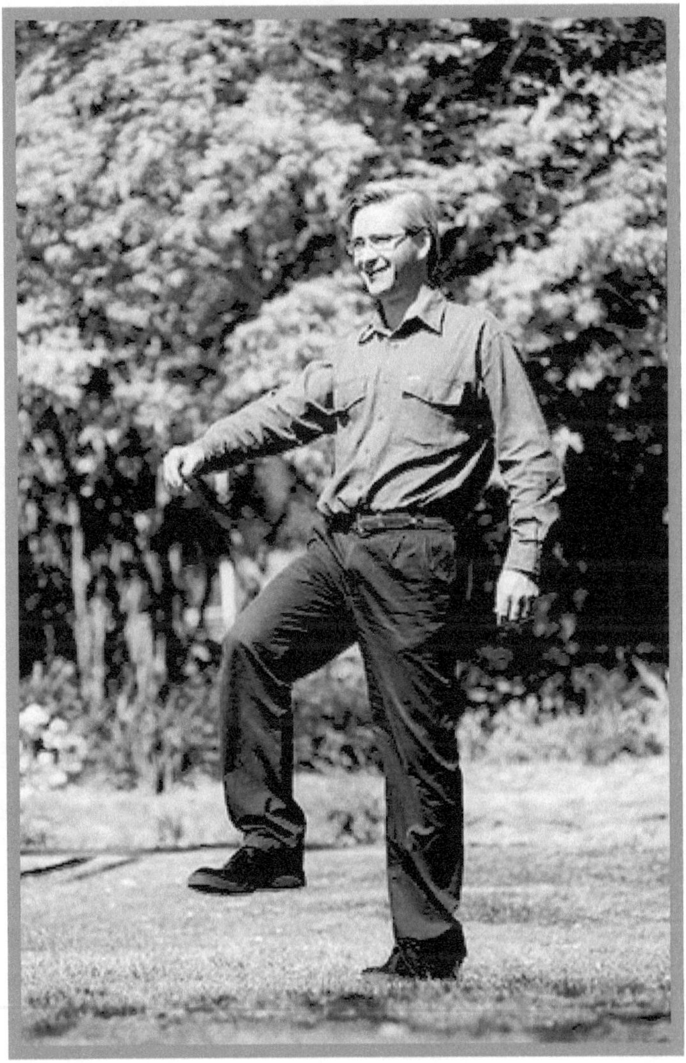

How does it feel?

Signs of good function include:

- ▶ Arms are loose;
- ▶ Arms swing freely from the shoulders;
- ▶ Movements are fluent;
- ▶ The arm and legs are synchronised.

Synchronisation is important here because it reflects the degree of coordination within one hemisphere. When you change from left arm and leg movement to right arm and leg movement it also requires a degree of synchronisation of right and left hemispheres. If the person can synchronise initially and then loses synchronisation this is a sign that same sided movement is stressful.

Watch for the following signs of stress:

1. Arms rigid and fists clenched;
2. Limited arm movement or arms swing only from elbow;
3. Limited leg movement;
4. Movements lack fluency;
5. Fists clenched;
6. Legs, arms or body rigid;
7. Legs and arms are out of synch;
8. Have them stop and restart again. Notice if there is any delay in starting.

Picture heading: **Signs of Stress**

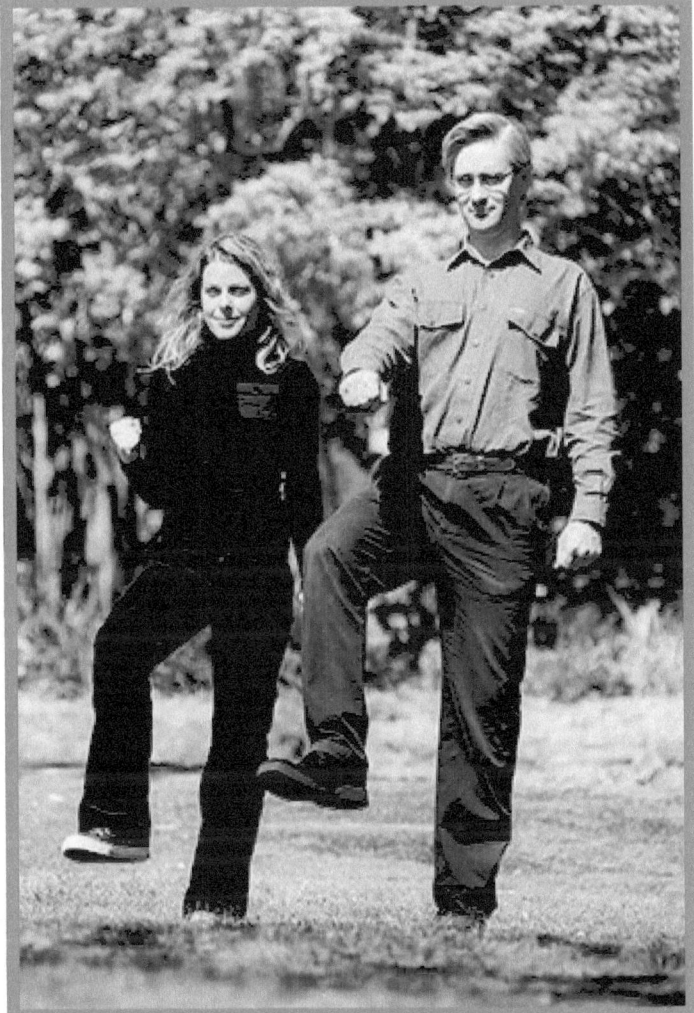

A number of signs of stress are displayed in the picture above:

▶ The woman is swinging her arm from the elbow rather than the shoulder;

▶ The man has a rigid body and his fists are clenched;

▶ The man's leg is splayed to the outside and thus not in alignment with the arm.

Give yourself a score out of 10 for your marching based on the following scale:

10 where there were no signs of stress;

8 if there is only one of the eight signs of stress from the table above

6 if there were two signs of stress from the table above

4 if there were three signs of stress from the table above

2 if there were four signs of stress from the table above

0 if there were five or more signs of stress from the table above

Your score here tells you something about the foundations upon which complex functions are built. People that have difficulty here often had stress in the initial stages of brain development (as infants). If you have a low score - do not worry – focus instead on how much better your brain will be able to function by the time you finish this book!

OPPOSITE SIDE MARCHING

The next step is to try marching like most people tend to walk and run, using the left arm and right leg or the right arm and left leg (see picture below).

Picture heading: **Opposite Side Marching**

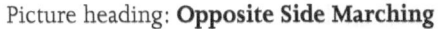

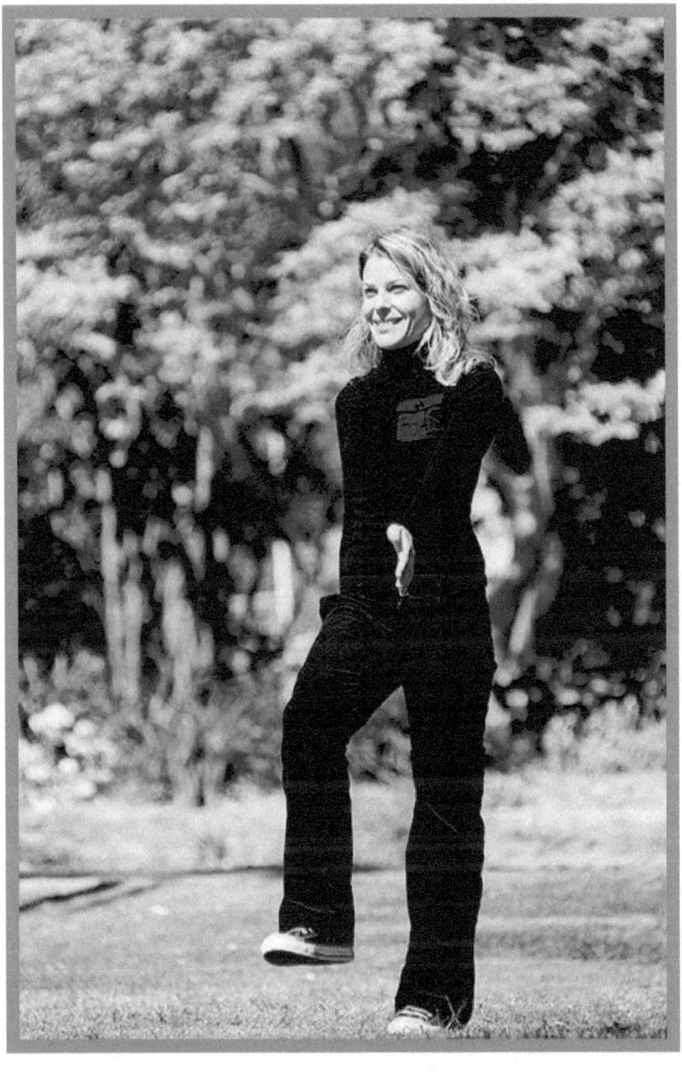

This type of marching has very different implications to same side marching. You may be good at one and poor at the other. It particularly relates to being able to put many things together – integrate a range of functions, as well as providing insight into how well the left and right hemispheres of the brain are able to coordinate.

Again note how it feels.

Signs of good function include:

- ▶ Arms are loose;
- ▶ Arms swing freely from the shoulders;
- ▶ Legs swing freely from the hips;
- ▶ Movements are fluent;
- ▶ The arm and legs are in synch.

Synchronisation is very important here as it is a sign that there is no delay in communication between the left and right hemispheres.

A lack of movement at both the hips and shoulders is an important sign that coordinated movement is stressful. A lot more coordination is needed for the arms to swing from the shoulders than from the elbow and for the legs to swing from the hips than from the knee1.

When people swing their arms from their elbow and knee rather than hips and shoulders it is a sign that, while they have a degree of coordination, coordination is stressful. So we use the degree of movement in the arms and legs as a barometer of the degree of stress in coordinating movement.

---

1 The reason for this is that there are many more senses (proprioceptors) in the hips and shoulders than in the elbow and knee, so movement at the shoulder and hip stimulates a great deal more brain activity than movement in the elbow and knee.

Picture heading: **Signs of Stress**

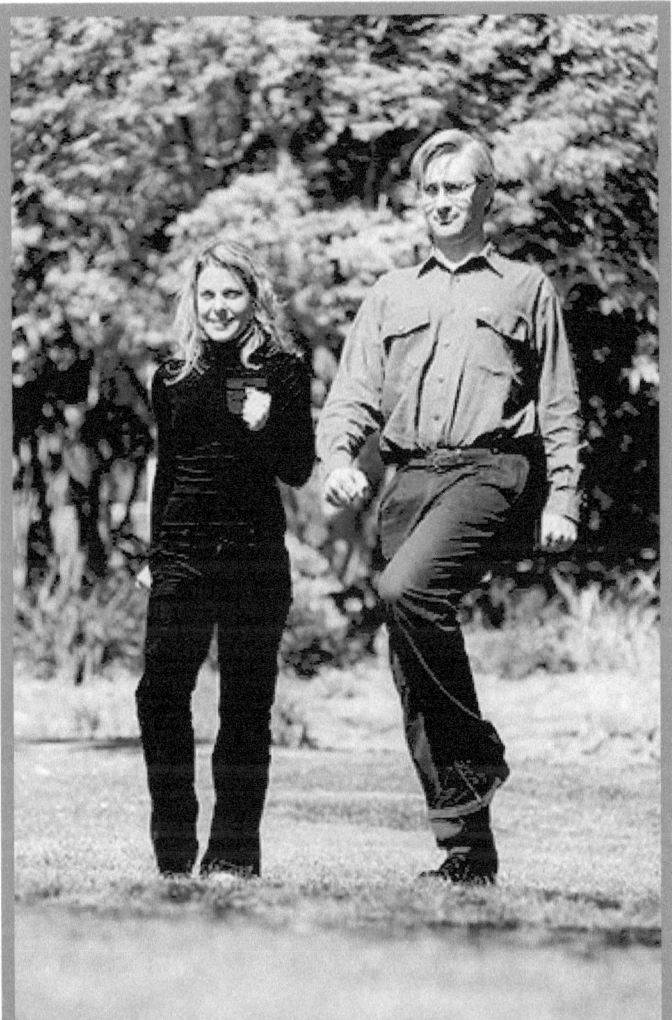

Signs of stress in the picture above include:

▶ The woman is swinging her arm from the elbow rather than the shoulder and has only a small degree of movement in the leg.

▶ The man has a very stiff body and clenched fists.

Picture heading: **Poor Synchronisation**

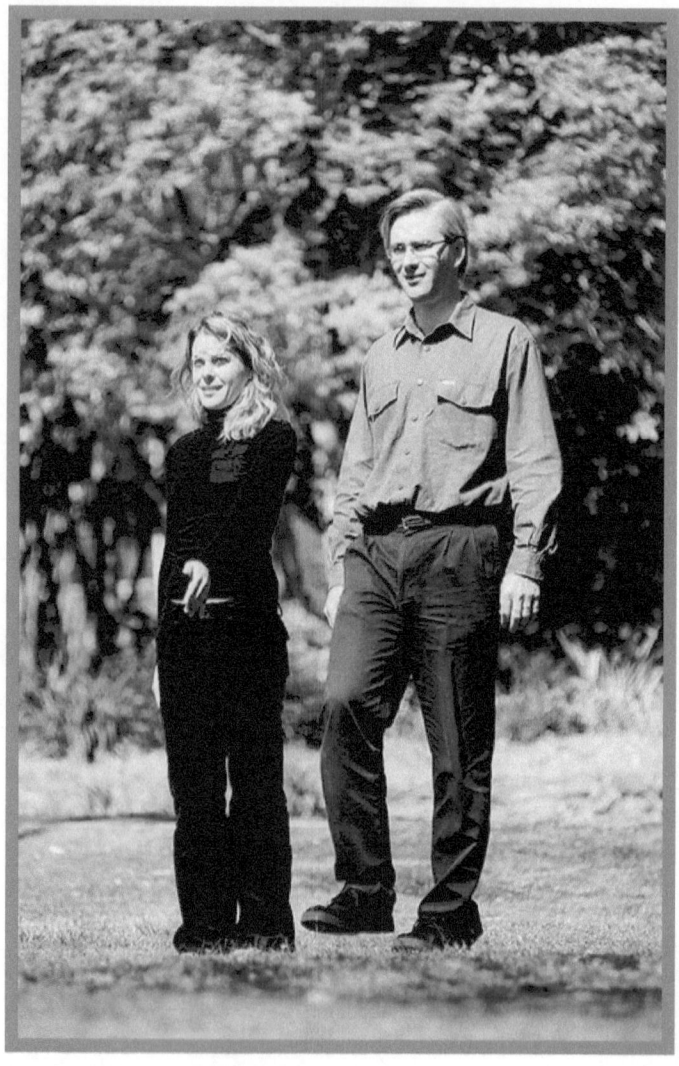

The above picture is taken at the beginning of the movement for both the woman and man. Notice how the woman has begun moving her hand but is yet to move her leg – which suggests that it is stressful to synchronise the movement of both arms and legs. The man has begun moving his leg before the arm has begun moving – again a sign of stress in synchronising movements.

To check for this lack of synchronisation watch your arm and leg carefully to see if one follows a little after the other. If there is good coordination and brain function both the arm and leg should move simultaneously.

Watch for the following signs of stress:

1. Arms rigid and fists clenched
2. Limited arm movement or arms swing only from elbow
3. Limited leg movement
4. Movements lack fluency
5. Fists clenched
6. Legs, arms or body rigid
7. Legs and arms are out of synch
8. Have them stop and restart again. Notice if there is any delay in starting.

Give yourself a score out of 10 for your marching based on the following scale:

10 where there were no signs of stress;

8 if there is only one of the eight signs of stress from the table above

6 if there were two signs of stress from the table above

4 if there were three signs of stress from the table above

2 if there were four signs of stress from the table above

0 if there were five or more signs of stress from the table above

If you have a low score - do not worry − focus instead on how much better your brain will be able to function by the time you finish this book!

BALANCE – STANDING STILL

Balance is very important for many day to day activities including walking and running, nearly any sporting activity, posture, many pain syndromes and nearly any physical activity.

The brain uses sight, mechanisms in the inner ear (vestibular) and feedback from muscles to help us to maintain balance. When these signals are out of synch or difficult for the brain to coordinate, we tend to be more readily motion sick.

The processing of signals from the inner ear is very important during early and later brain development. These signals are used a great deal by the brain to coordinate physical activity. Anyone who has had an inner ear infection can testify to how debilitating it is to have this sense disturbed.

Our ability to balance has wider implications for our health than just being important for movement. Problems with physical balance also tend to occur during times when we feel "off balance", "ungrounded", or "off centre" in life. These emotional states can affect balance and poor physical balance can also affect how we feel.

The simplest way to test for balance is to stand on one leg. Make sure the legs are not touching.

1. First stand on one leg for 10 seconds.
2. Then stand on the other leg for 10 seconds.
3. Continue standing on one leg and close your eyes (balance for 10 seconds).
4. Swap to the other leg, balance and then close your eyes (balance for 10 seconds).

Picture heading: **Balance – eyes open and closed**

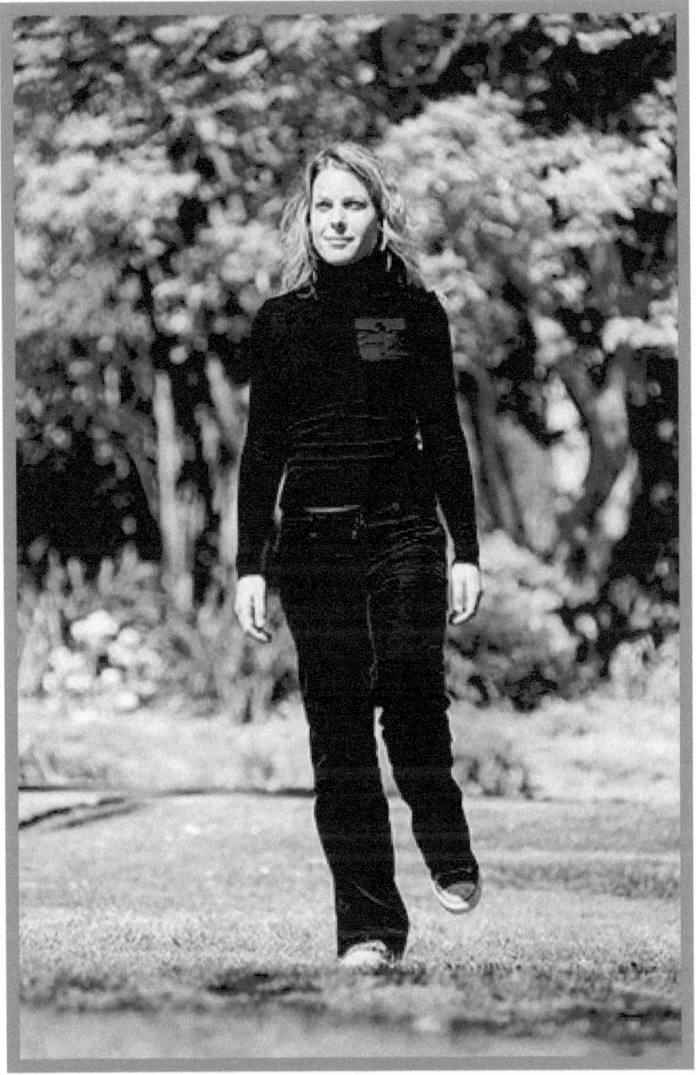

How easy was it to stand on one leg?

If you have good balance you should be able to stand on one leg without a great deal of movement for 10 seconds with eyes shut.

Give yourself a score out of 10 for your balance based on the following scale:

> 10 where you could stand comfortably eyes open and shut for 10 seconds;
>
> 8 if you could stand comfortably eyes open for 10 seconds but wobbled and moved while standing eyes shut for 10 seconds
>
> 6 if you could stand 10 seconds eyes open but only stand eyes shut for 6-9 seconds
>
> 4 if you could stand 10 seconds eyes open but only stand eyes shut for 3-6 seconds
>
> 2 if you could stand only 7 seconds eyes open and had difficulty eyes closed
>
> 0 if could stand less than 7 seconds eyes open and had difficulty eyes closed

So your score here is important not just as a sign of your physical stability but also because it is an indicator of emotional balance as well. The difference between eyes open and shut is that you can only use your vestibular (inner ear) sense when your eyes are shut. When your eyes are open you can use your sight and vestibular to help you to balance. If the vestibular is not working well it will be considerably more difficult to stand with your eyes shut.

WALK THE TIGHTROPE

There are two mechanisms within the inner ear that provide information for balance. The first tells the brain where the head is when it is held still. It acts a little like a carpenter's level – telling the brain what angle the head is being held at. This was the mechanism we assessed when you stood still on one leg.

The second mechanism responds to movement of the head, helping the brain to balance while the head is in motion (dynamic balance).

To test for dynamic balance, imagine you are walking a tightrope. Have one foot placed immediately in front of the other so the back of one foot just touches the toes of the other. Walk slowly by placing the back foot in front of the other foot, just like you would if you were walking a tightrope.

Picture heading: **Walk the tightrope - eyes open and closed**

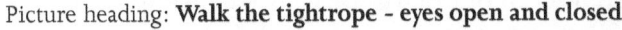

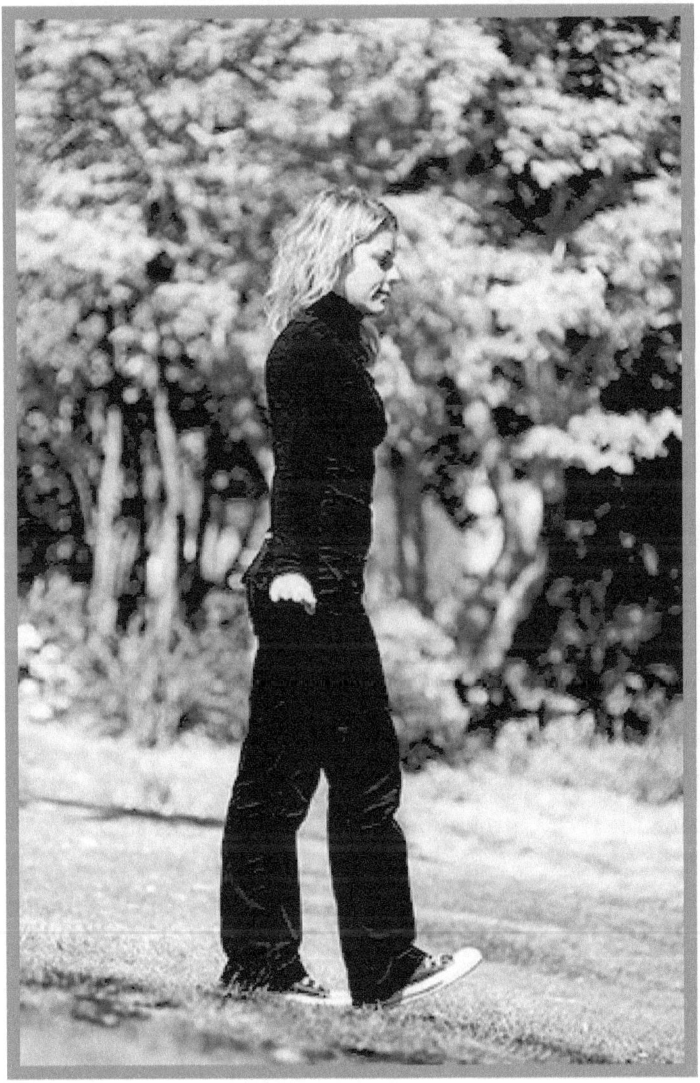

Once you have walked 10 metres turn and do it again but with eyes shut.

How easy was it to walk the tightrope?

If you have good balance you should be able to walk slowly in one line without wobbling or overbalancing.

Give yourself a score out of 10 for your balance based on the following scale:

10 where you could walk in a straight line comfortably eyes open and shut for 10 metres;

8 if you could walk for 10 metres eyes open and closed but wobbled significantly;

6 if you could walk eyes shut only 6 metres without falling over

4 if you could walk eyes open but could not walk with eyes shut more than 5metres

2 if you could walk with eyes open only 6 metres and could not walk well eyes shut

0 if you could not walk eyes open 6 metres without overbalancing

Dynamic balance is very important for movement and physical coordination. It also often relates to how we respond to change. Do we keep our centre as we move forward and change? The difference between eyes open and shut is that you can only use your vestibular (inner ear) sense when eyes are shut. If this sense of balance is not working well it will be considerably more difficult to walk with your eyes shut.

HEARING

Hearing is one of the earliest senses to operate and is very important for brain development and later function.

Even when people can hear perfectly, they may be distracted or stressed by certain sounds, over-react to loud noises and/or have difficulty comprehending the meaning of sounds.

In this section you can assess your own hearing and auditory comprehension, or have someone read a couple of paragraphs of a book and then quiz you about what they read.

Signs of stress with hearing and auditory comprehension include:

1. Are you oversensitive to sounds?
2. Do you get easily startled by loud sounds?
3. Do certain sounds annoy you?
4. Do you hear and understand the words in songs?
5. Can you listen and respond in a discussion of a large group of people;
6. Are you easily distracted?
7. Do you understand what people say the first time they say it?
8. Do you understand the nuances of what people say including the tone they use?

Score yourself out of 10. If many of the signs of stress above apply to you then the score should be low. If only one factor applies but it is quite severe score yourself 5 or less depending on the severity. To score above 7, two factors or less should apply and neither should be severe.

READING

Reading is so important in modern life, and yet few people realise how complex the process of reading is. Reading involves a number of areas of the brain coordinating so that you can decode the words and understand what you read. It is a complex brain function that requires good communication between many areas of the brain.

In this section you can assess your own reading, or you can read a couple of paragraphs of a book and have someone quiz you about them.

Signs of stress with reading include:

1. Do you get tired reading?
2. Do you understand what you read the first time you read it or do you need to re-read a section in order to comprehend its meaning?
3. Do you find it difficult to comprehend what you read even if you re-read the section?
4. Do you read at the same pace or slower than you speak? (note: a good reader reads much faster than they can speak)
5. Is it hard to keep focussed on what you read?
6. Do your eyes get tired when you read or do you get headaches when you read?
7. When you read to yourself do you still mouth the words to yourself or do you just see the words?

If you have better comprehension reading out loud it is likely that your auditory comprehension is better than your visual comprehension. This often occurs where the client has so much difficulty decoding words that the brain ends up paying little attention to the meaning of words being read. This can be partly a result of the mind getting bored with waiting for the word to be decoded. When it is read aloud the client hears the story, and the mind takes in the meaning as it hears the words.

Score yourself out of 10. If many of the signs of stress above apply to you then the score should be low. If only one factor applies but it is quite severe score yourself 5 or less depending on the severity. To score above 7, two factors or less should apply and neither should be severe.

CONCENTRATION

I would now like you to assess your normal level of concentration.

Are you able to sit down and apply yourself to a mental task for an hour without your mind wondering?

Are you able to sit and listen to someone giving a lecture without your mind wondering every couple of minutes?

Score yourself out of 10. A mark of 7 or more indicates that you can concentrate well at all times. A mark around 5 indicates that you can sometimes concentrate well. A mark around 3 indicates that it is always difficult to concentrate.

SPEECH

I would now like you to assess your speech. Do you stutter or have difficulty expressing yourself to other people? Is it difficult to speak clearly?

Score yourself out of 10. A mark of 7 indicates that you occasionally have difficulty expressing yourself to other people, particularly under stress. A mark of 5 indicates that you stutter occasionally. A mark of 3 indicates you stutter one syllable in ten. A mark of 1 indicates you stutter one syllable in four.

ADDING UP YOUR ASSESSMENT

Add up the scores from your assessment:	
Same side marching	10
Opposite side marching	10
Balance – standing	10
Walking the tightrope	10
Hearing	10
Reading	10
Concentrating	10
Speech	10
Total	**80**

APPLYING THE POWER TOOLS

We will apply our power tools in a sequence that helps to improve overall function and communication first before we consider specific areas such as reading or vision. Why? Because if you have difficulty with overall function then you are likely to have poor brain function in the specific areas as well.

To improve overall function we will first focus on coordinated movement. Establishing good movement and coordination lays a foundation for other complex tasks. Good builders always make sure they lay good solid foundations. It is the same with brain function.

You will get the best results if you complete Step 2 in the order outlined below.

1. SAME SIDE MARCHING

Our aim here is to be able to do same side marching with no signs of stress – that is a perfect score of 10 or at least a score of 8 before moving on.

Same side marching is important because it provides an indication of how solid the building blocks of learning – the primitive reflexes - have been integrated.

Infants have reflexes that help them perform certain functions. These 'primitive" reflexes are useful to a point but need to be inhibited as the next stage of development takes place. If they are not inhibited then the more complex reflexes will not be able to take over and coordination will be impaired.

There are a range of primitive reflexes and they affect a wide range of functions. For example if you touch a baby's palm its fist will clench – this enables it to grip. However, if an adult has this reflex then writing becomes very difficult because it is difficult to grip the pen between the thumb and index finger without activating the palm reflex.

We will not consider all the reflexes here but keep in mind that if you still have difficulties with same side marching after you do the processes in this section then it would be advisable to seek help from a qualified Holistic Kinesiologist or primitive reflex therapist.

When working in clinic on same sided marching I often assess and address individual primitive reflexes first, and then move on to focus on same sided movements. In this book we will start in a similar way – focussing on a simple way of activating one of the more important reflexes, the startle reflex before moving on to same sided movements.

Startle

When startled, babies will breathe in and throw their arms and legs backwards. This section will be particularly useful for you if you are easily startled, or if you have a tendency under stress to withdraw physically and/or emotionally.

Start with yourself rolled into a ball. To activate the reflex breathe in sharply and simultaneously extend your legs and arms back quickly (straightening from the ball and getting to a point where your spine arches backwards). Hold your breath out (for 2 or 3 seconds) and then hold the acupoint GV16 on the back of your skull (see diagram below). If possible have someone else hold the point and wait until you feel a deep sense of peace.

"Beginning"

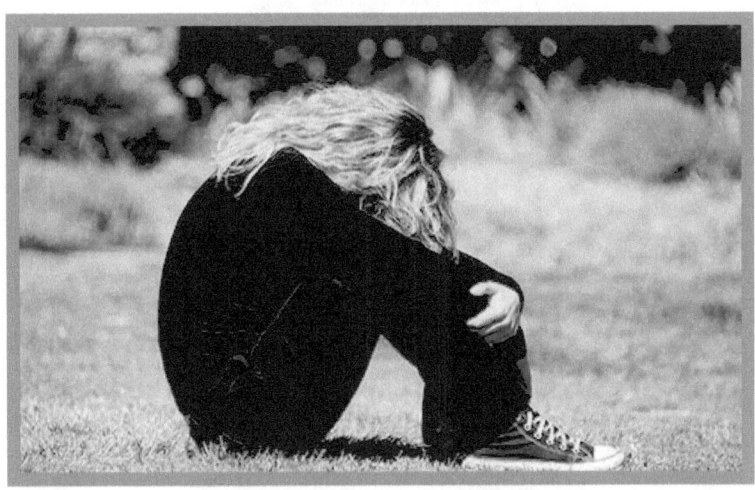

"End"

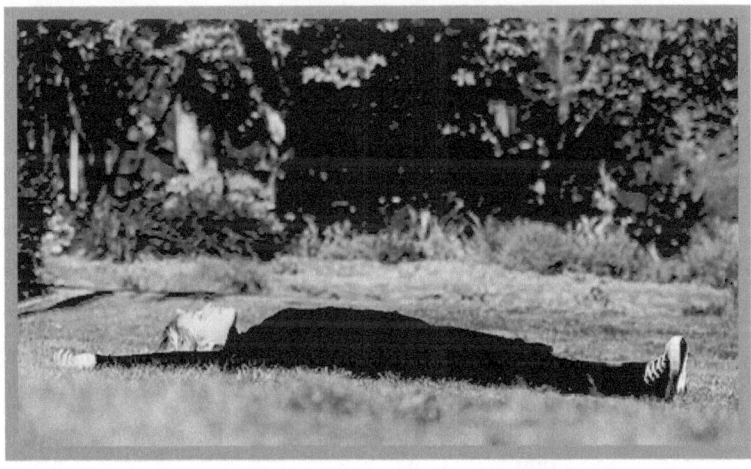

You may need to hold the point for some time – 30 minutes to an hour depending on how much stress this pattern activates.

Once you finish, try activating the reflex again and see if it feels different. Changing this startle response can make a massive difference to your life, not just in terms of brain function but how you interact in life.

Governing 16

Governing 16 (Gv16) "Palace of Wind"

Located on the base of the skull (occiput) in the depression immediately below the bump on the back of the skull.

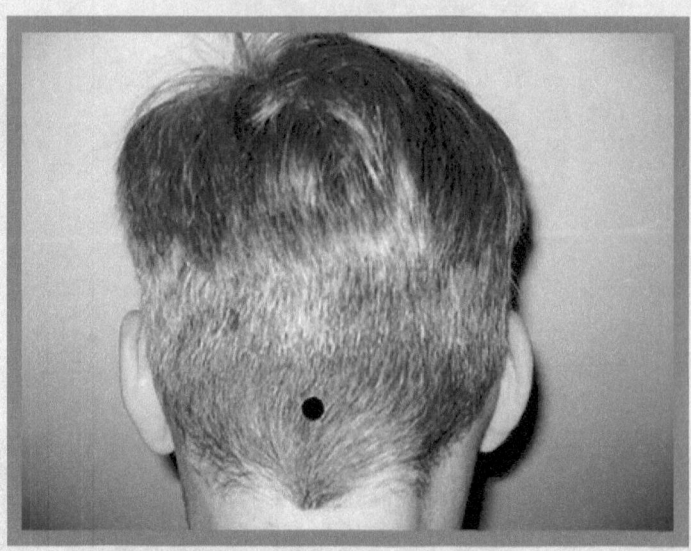

The Governing vessel is extremely important for brain function. This point is particularly useful because the Governing vessel plunges deeply into the brain from this point. This point directly links with many aspects of the physical brain.

The name of the point refers to wind. The Chinese use the term wind to describe a certain type of qi movement (movement of the energy of the body). Just like wind in nature is responsible for movement, wind in the body promotes movement. This movement may become problematic, just like a strong wind in nature can cause havoc. Wind is particularly important for brain function. Perverse wind can cause a range of symptoms including dizziness, headaches, and confusion.

Gv16 is very useful for calming wind and bringing calm to the mind.

GV16 is near the base of the brain and relates particularly to:

- ✓ Survival functions (automatic reactions to potential threats);
- ✓ Responses to fear;
- ✓ Balance;
- ✓ Vision;
- ✓ Smell;
- ✓ Taste.

From a Western neurology perspective Gv16 can be used to reduce stress in the brain stem and limbic centres of the brain.

MARCHING

Try same sided marching while someone holds the Bladder 9 acupoints on the back of your skull (see diagram below). Alternatively you could lie down on a bed, hold the points on the back of your head as you raise one leg and arm (on the same side of the body).

Bladder 9

Bladder 9 (Bl9) "Jade Pillow"

Located on the back of the head, about 1½ thumb widths out from the bump at the back of the head.

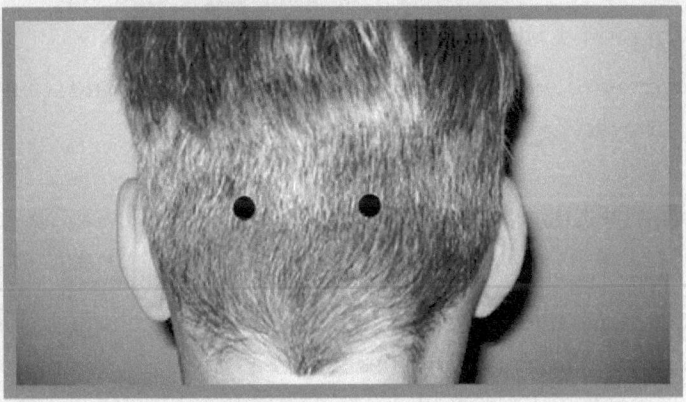

It is an important point for influencing the functions of the cerebellum (sometimes called the second brain or little brain) that is a very important part of the brain for coordinating fine motor movement. This point also addresses our survival reactions and emotions.

Bl9 improves fine motor control (activities such as writing and speech) and dizziness. This point has also been traditionally used for vision and smell.

Reassess

Get up and have a walk around for a couple of minutes, swinging your arms freely.

Try same side marching. Assess your score out of 10. If you score 8/10 or better move on to the next stage.

If it is not instantly improved it either means:

▶ you need to hold the points for longer (try holding the points a little longer);

▶ you need to give the brain time to integrate the changes (if you give yourself at least a week break before coming back and reassessing your same side marching – you may find it has improved substantially after one or two weeks);

▶ you need more work on the primitive reflexes (and would benefit from seeing a qualified practitioner).

2. OPPOSITE SIDE MARCHING

Reassess your opposite side marching. It may be different after having worked on same side marching. Often it improves although sometimes it seems worse. The reason it can seem worse is that your opposite side marching may have been built on a poor foundation. When you readjust the foundations by working on same side marching and reflexes, it can take a while for the brain to readjust. It may need to unwind the old compensated pattern of opposite side marching and start afresh with a more natural pattern of marching.

Commando Crawl

The next step is to start with the first type of crawling we learn – belly crawling or commando crawl.

Lie on your stomach and start crawling with your belly on the ground (see picture).

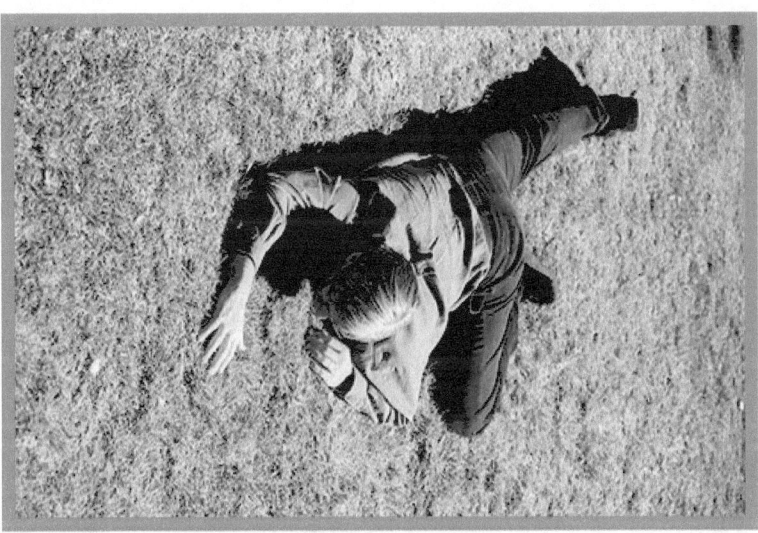

You may have difficulty crawling. Signs of stress are shown in the picture below.

▶ Notice the man's leg does not move as far out to the side, his right arm is not extended far in front of him and he is trying to lift off the floor.

▶ The woman is shuffling without moving her legs at the hips.

33

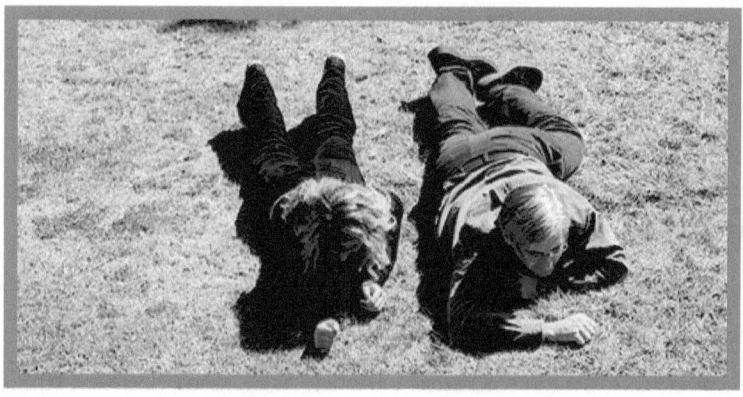

If it is not completely fluent then stop with each movement and hold or have someone hold the Bladder 62 points on the outside of the ankle in the diagram below. You may need to hold the points for some time. Move again and hold the points. Keep doing this until the movement becomes more fluent.

Bladder 62

Bladder 62 (Bl62) "Extending vessel"

Located in the depression below the middle of the ankle on the outside of the foot.

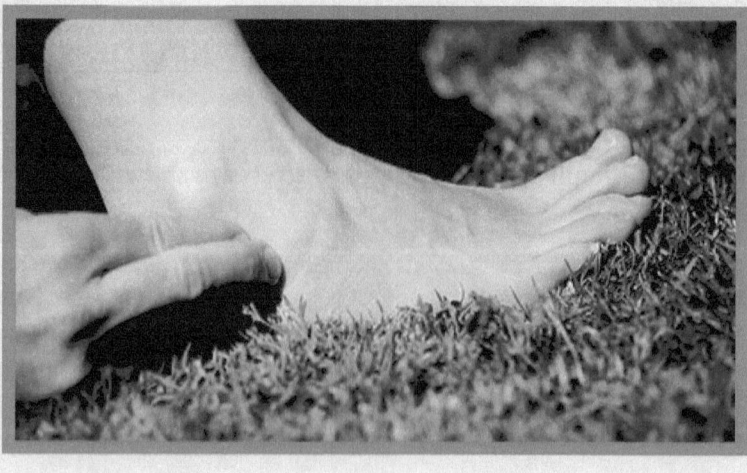

The name of Bl62 relates to the ability of the body to move (extend and flex). It relates to all the musculature. The link with extension/contraction relates it directly to walking and ability to coordinate muscles.

Bl62 is the key point for reducing stress in the communication pathways of the brain – the commissural fibres, association and projection fibres. It also can be taken to relate to the communication between the deep brain centres and outer cortex, the front and back and the top and bottom of the brain.

It also has a role to play in wakefulness and alertness.

Bl62 is a very important point for addressing internal links within the brain. It relates particularly to:

- ✓ Left and right confusion;
- ✓ Reasoning through emotional confusion;
- ✓ Epilepsy;
- ✓ Insomnia;
- ✓ Alertfulness, wakefulness;
- ✓ Walking gait and leg muscle tone;
- ✓ Headache;
- ✓ Hearing;
- ✓ Vision.

Hands and Knees Crawl

Now try crawling on your hands and knees. Again if you lack fluency stop and hold the point below the ankle at each stage of the movement until the movement becomes fluent.

Marching

Try marching with opposite arm and leg. If there are signs of stress hold the points on the ankle (Bladder 62) until you feel totally relaxed and at peace.

March again and reassess. If the marching is not totally fluent try marching while someone holds the points at the back of your head (Gv16 and/or Bl9).

Reassess

Get up and have a walk around for a couple of minutes, swinging your arms freely.

Try opposite side marching. Assess your score out of 10. If you score 8/10 or better move on to the next stage.

From here on you can turn to the function that you scored lowest on in the assessment. Once that function improves move on to any other functions that need improvement.

If it is not instantly improved it either means:

▶ you need to hold the points for longer (try holding the points a little longer);

▶ you need to give the brain time to integrate the changes (if you give yourself at least a week break before coming back and reassessing your marching – you may find it has improved substantially after one or two weeks).

3. BALANCE – STANDING STILL

Re-assess how well you can balance. It may well have improved now that you have improved your coordinated movement.

If you are still shaky with eyes open, balance on one foot eyes open while someone holds a point on the back of your head (either Bl9 or Gv16 in the diagram below – for a description of these points turn back to the section on same sided marching).

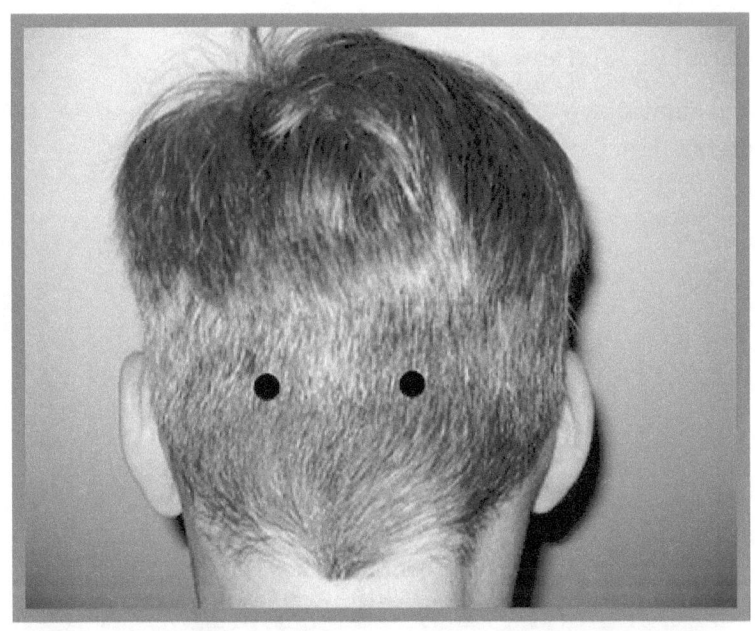

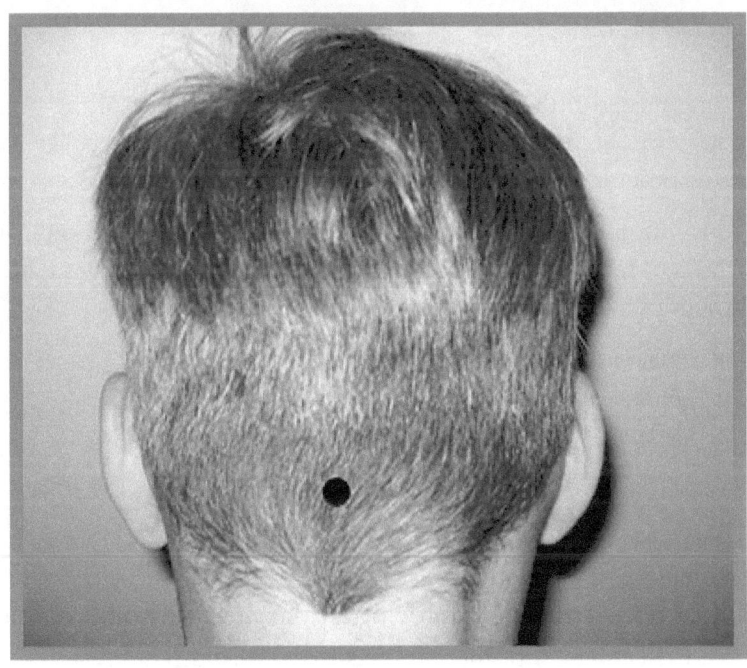

Bladder 10

Bladder 10 (Bl10) "Heavenly Pillar"

Located immediately below the base of the occiput around 1½ thumb widths out from the vertebra of the neck.

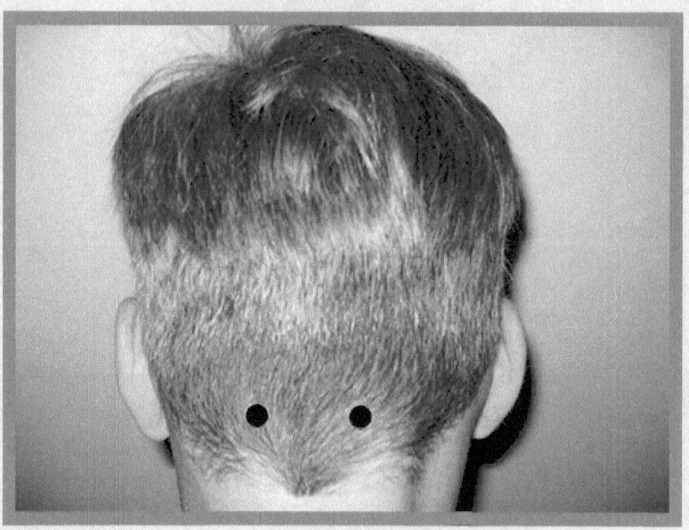

The name relates to the position of the point on the back of the occiput – the head can be seen as representing heaven and the body is like earth, hence the point is the pillar on which the head (heaven) rests.

Bl10 is an important point for reducing stress associated with coordinating fine motor movement and balance (particularly in the region of the cerebellum part of the brain). It is a very important point for:

- ✓ Vision;
- ✓ Fine motor movement and cerebellum;
- ✓ Balance and dizziness;
- ✓ Headaches;
- ✓ Confusion.

If it does not seem to be improving try the alternate points on the back of the head (Bladder 10 points on the second diagram below).

Once you can stand with eyes open try standing on one foot with eyes closed. If you are still shaky have someone hold the first set of points on the back of your head (Gv16 and Bl9). If it does not seem to be improving try the alternate points on the back of the head (Bl10 see diagram above).

4. WALKING THE TIGHT ROPE

Re-assess how well you can walk the tight rope. It may well have improved now that you have worked on movement and static balance.

If you still have difficulty with eyes open, try moving slowly with eyes open while someone holds the points on the back of your head used in the previous section (GV16 and Bl9). If it does not seem to be improving try the other point on the back of the head used in the previous section (Bl10).

Once you can move with eyes open try moving with eyes closed. If you still have difficulty have someone hold the same points on the back of your head.

If it is very difficult to balance while someone holds the points, try lying or sitting down while the points are held, and then recheck your balance again.

5. READING

Reassess your reading. If your eyes still feel strained or get tired then hold the points immediately below the eyes (Stomach 1) in the diagram below. These points are great for any eye or vision related problem.

Stomach 1

Stomach 1 (St1) "Container of Tears"

Located immediately below the eyes on the edge of the bone that surrounds the eye.

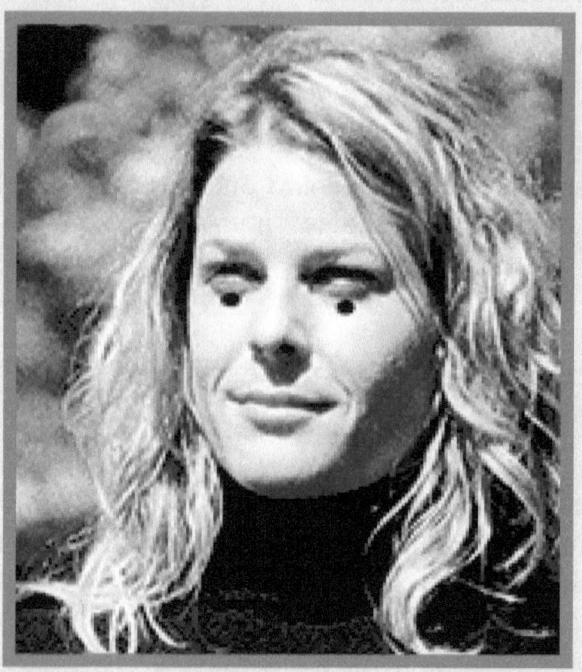

It is commonly used in Chinese Medicine for treating a wide range of eye and vision conditions including:

Redness, swelling and pain of the eyes,

- ✓ Watery eyes;
- ✓ Obstruction of vision;
- ✓ Dimness of vision;
- ✓ Short sightedness;
- ✓ Visual dizziness;
- ✓ Night blindness;
- ✓ Itching of the eyes;
- ✓ Twitching of the eyelids.

If you are having difficulty understanding and remembering what you read hold the points on the back of your head near the mastoid process (Gall Bladder 20 in the diagram below). These points on the back of the skull help with seeing things clearly and understanding what we see.

Gall Bladder 20

Gall Bladder 20 (GB20) "Wind Pool"

Located below the occiput (back of the skull) midway to the ear in a depression formed between where the two major muscles of the neck attach to the skull (if you move your head to the side and forwards and backwards you should be able to feel the ends of these muscles).

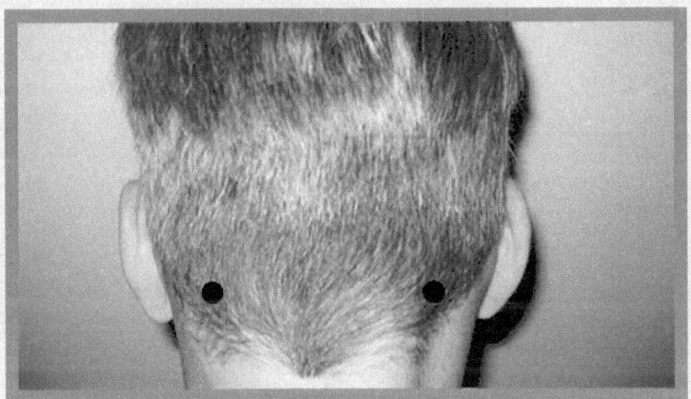

GB20 is an extremely important point for headaches of all kinds. Located on the occiput it is also a key point for eyes.

It is commonly used to improve:

- ✓ Vision;
- ✓ Balance and dizziness;
- ✓ Smell;
- ✓ Hearing;
- ✓ Sluggish thinking;
- ✓ Clarity of thinking and comprehension;
- ✓ Memory;
- ✓ Speech.

Keep holding these points until the reading improves. If comprehension is still difficult also try Gv16 (see description in same side marching section) on the back of the head and Bl62 (see description in the opposite side marching section) on the outside of the ankle.

4. HEARING

There are some wonderful points for all aspects of hearing. My favourite is called listening palace, and it is on the front of the ear in the dent where the jaw connects with the skull.

If you have difficulties with sensitivity to noise have someone make a lot of noise while you hold these points near your ears. If you have problems with a particular type of sound have someone make that sound while you hold the points.

Eventually you should find the noises become much less distressing.

If you have difficulties with comprehension, try to make out the words as you listen to songs while you hold the points.

Small Intestine 19

Small Intestine 19 (SI19) "Listening Palace"

Located just in front of the ear in the depression that is formed when you open your mouth (between the ear and the tempero-mandibular joint).

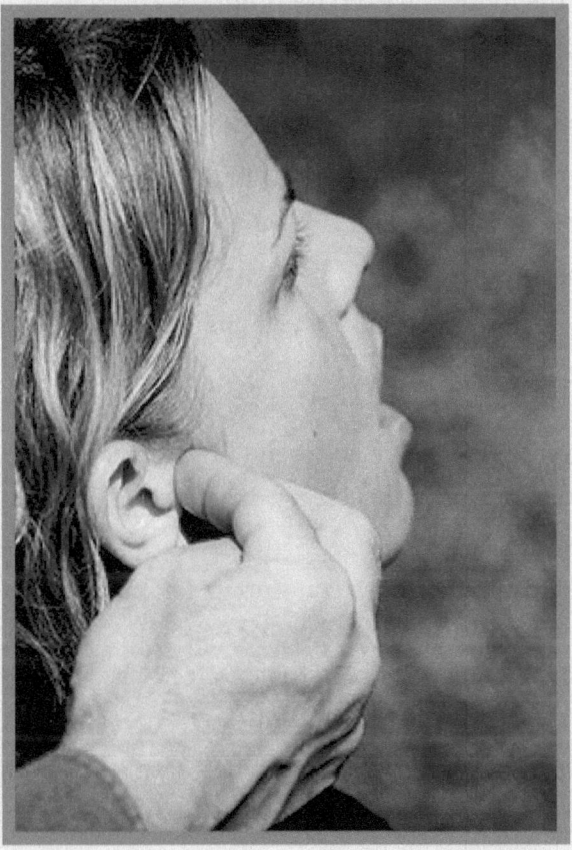

The acupuncture system actually enters the ear from this point, so it is very commonly used for improving ear conditions and hearing including:

- ✓ Deafness;
- ✓ Tinnitus;
- ✓ Discharge from the ear;
- ✓ Circulation within the inner ear.

5. FOCUS AND MEMORY

The best way to improve focus is to train your mind to be receptive to the outside world. The Chinese say we are most receptive when we are empty. Memory is also improved when we are able to fully focus and absorb.

I have found the following exercise produces amazing results when it is practiced every day. It has many effects including:

- ▶ Improving acceptance;
- ▶ Improving concentration and focus;
- ▶ Sharpens our hearing;
- ▶ Improves memory;
- ▶ Allows us to absorb more and remember more easily;
- ▶ Calms and relaxes.

I have never known anyone that did not improve their concentration dramatically that practiced this exercise regularly.

I did this exercise every day for three years and by the end of that period I found that my ability to concentrate for long periods was amazing. I remember sitting in lectures for three days in a row without losing concentration once, and later being able to recall everything that was said. I had never experienced anything like it.

It also helped me to deal with my wife's severe illness, inducing calm and acceptance.

Listening to Sound Exercise

This exercise can be done inside or outside. It is best done where you can hear the sounds of birds and animals or at least the sounds of traffic passing by irregularly. This exercise is done for a minimum of 10 minutes, preferably 20 minutes. Initially the time will seem to drag, but after a week or two your ability to concentrate will improve and the time will flash by like a blink of an eye.

Sit with your back against a wall with your legs out in front of you. Place a pillow behind to support your lumber spine and ensure your back is straight. Make sure you are comfortable.

Take three deep breaths. Begin to hear all the sounds that are around you. I want you to pick out one sound that is irregular and infrequent. Focus on this sound. It may be the call of a bird or the passing of a car. If your mind wanders bring it back listening for the sound. After a while if you are able to hold concentration on that sound widen your awareness and allow all the sounds to wash over you. Imagine the sounds are like water from the ocean washing over you, a rock. You do not think about or analyse the sounds, just witness them. Allow them to flood over you.

After twenty minutes bring your mind back to centre, take three deep breaths and stretch and rise.

Drive and Determination

Concentration and drive often go hand in hand. Poor concentration can be caused by lack of drive and application as well as excessive drive and application. Excessive drive affects concentration because it depletes the body and affects the spirit.

There is a point that helps balance drive. It relates directly to will power, the ability to unrelentingly pursue a given course. It is called the "room of will" (Bladder 52) – see diagram below.

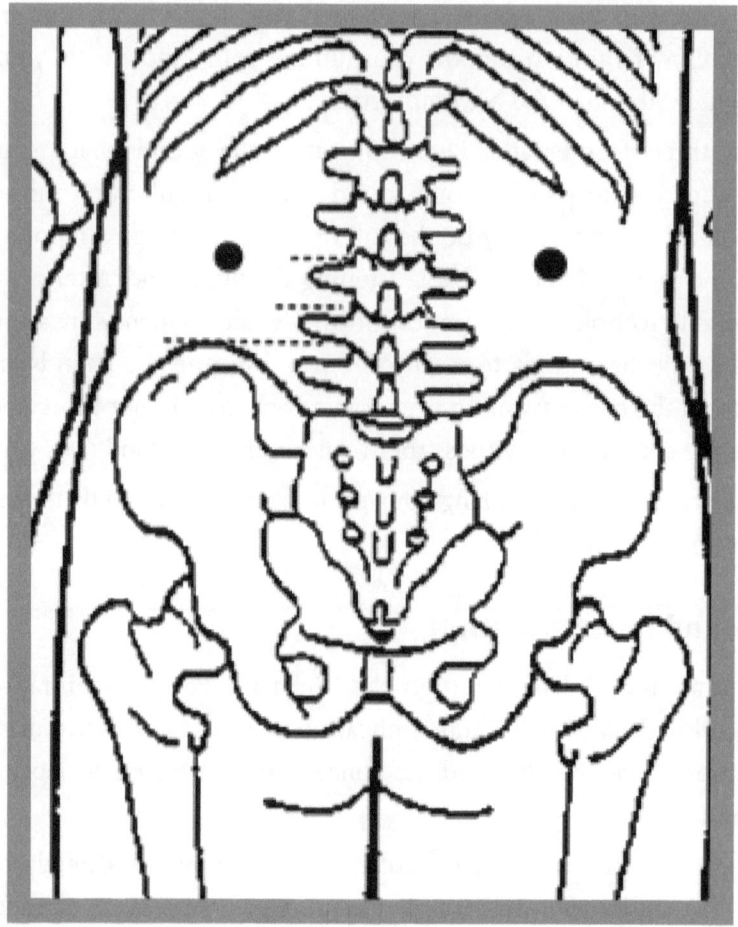

It is found on the back, the width of your hand (ie little finger to index finger - about 6cm on an adult) out from the second lumbar vertebra. If you follow the bottom of your ribcage around to the back it will lead you to the last thoracic vertebra. The second lumbar vertebra is two vertebra down from there. The lumbar vertebra feel more rounded than the pointy thoracic vertebra so if you trace down the spine you should be able to find the first lumbar vertebra by feeling for where the spine is less pointy. It can help to have the back arched.

Hold this point while you visualise the following:

> *Under-active will: Imagine being able to do what is most important for you in your life in the way that you want. Imagine achieving what is most important to you.*
>
> *Overactive will: Imagine feeling like you are heading in the direction of your choice, flowing with the tide of life like a river through rambling hills. As you flow along feel the joy of feeling free to just go with the flow and live your truth. Allow yourself to be diverted around obstacles, at peace knowing that you still have a firm idea of where you are eventually heading and understanding that each diversion provides an opportunity for a different view of your path and thus an opportunity for further learning and enjoyment.*

An Open Heart and Memory

Memory improves when we are focussed, open and more aware of our surroundings. It also improves when we are internally open to our heart and not seeking to hide from our past.

In Chinese medicine there are three major causes of poor memory:

- ▶ A disturbed spirit – usually due to a trauma that has resulted in us shutting down;
- ▶ Poor vitality – when the body is ill or our reserves are low our memory suffers;
- ▶ Anxiety and tension that affects our ability to relax and let go.

Memory involves a process of letting go and opening up internally. There are a number of points that help with this process. My favourite for promoting greater inner connection is "Inner Pass" (Pericardium 6) a point in the middle of the inner aspect of the arm around two thumb widths from the wrist crease (see diagram below).

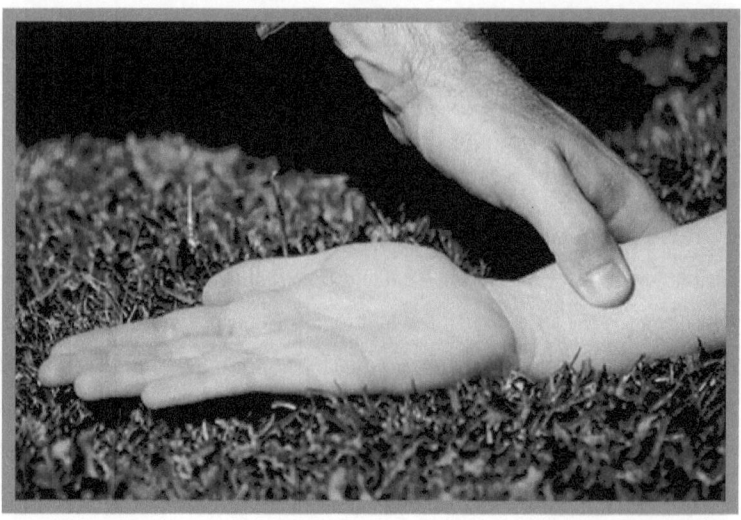

When you hold this point, allow yourself to relax and try the following visualisation:

Focus on your heart. As you look closer you can see a tiny door in the middle of the heart. This is the doorway to your heart of hearts, your core feelings, the core you. This door may have been shut for a long time. It may be that you shut the door in response to some hurt. Understand that by shutting the door you locked your spontaneous and joyful self away, effectively locking in the hurt. When you are ready allow the door to open and your heart of hearts to infuse into your whole being, no longer held captive and suppressed behind your own barriers. It infuses you with the joy of the child, the wonder of life, spontaneity and love.

6. Speech

Speech is affected by a range of factors. It is influenced by internal confidence and our ability to comfortably put ourselves forward. How well do we assert ourselves in our life? The mind has to function well to speak. Speech involves:

▶ Choosing the right words;

▶ Using tone for emphasis and to generate understanding;

▶ Careful coordination of many muscles in the mouth and throat;

▶ Use of the lungs and diaphragm.

Hold the Governing 15 point at the back of your head while you speak. If it is more difficult to speak well in certain circumstances, eg in front of a group of people, try to recreate those circumstances while you hold the point or at least imagine yourself in those circumstances while you hold the point.

You may need to hold the point for some time. If you are by yourself try reading out loud while you hold the point. If you are still not speaking fluently either hold the point for longer or alternatively you may hold Gall Bladder 20 (refer to the section on reading for a description of the point).

Governing Vessel 15

Governing Vessel 15 (GV15) " Gate of Muteness"

Located in the depression on the middle of the neck just below the occiput (skull) and just above the first vertebra you can feel in the neck (C2).

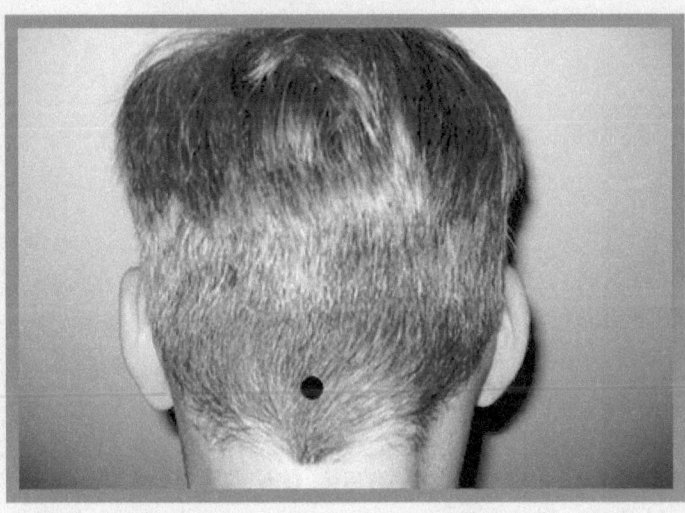

This is the key point for all speech problems including the loudness of the voice, the ability to articulate well and to choose words cleverly.

Traditional indications for this point include:

- ✓ stiffness of the tongue with inability to speak;
- ✓ loss of voice;
- ✓ flaccidity of the tongue;
- ✓ brain confusion.

STEP 3

REASSESS AND SCORE

Now it is time to reassess your function and find your new score. Typically you could expect to have improved substantially in a number of areas. If there is more to be done I would suggest you either spend more time in particular areas or see a qualified Holistic Kinesiologist who can find and defuse the missing links.

STEP 4

REINFORCEMENT

A range of exercises can help reinforce the changes made as a result of the work in this book.

If you had difficulty with marching, I suggest you crawl for 5 minutes a day for 3 or 4 weeks. This will reinforce the pathways for coordinated movement in your brain.

If you had difficulty with balance, meditation and breathing exercises can help to keep you centred and balanced. You could try the listening to sound exercise in the focus section as an exercise to keep you centred.

If you had difficulty with reading, it might be worthwhile to repeat the reading section again in a few months time, to see if you can diffuse more stress.

For focus and memory the consistent practice of the listening to sound exercise will make a major difference over time.

USING BRAIN POWER TO HELP COMMON CONDITIONS

Condition	What to do	Points to use
Poor coordination	Improve same sided marching first then opposite side marching	Same sided marching – Gv16 and Bl9; opposite side Bl62 (can also try Gv16 and Bl9)
Poor balance	Balance - standing still and walking the tightrope eyes open and closed	Bl10 and Bl9
Reading	Improve coordination and balance first then improve eye function and comprehension	Eye function – St1 Comprehension – GB20 Extra points to try – Gv16 and Bl62
Hearing	Improve coordination and balance first then hold hearing points while making noise	SI19
Vision	Improve coordination and balance first and then hold vision points while looking in different directions	St1 and GB20 Bl9, Bl10 and GV16 can also be used to improve vision
Sensitive to touch, dislike of being touched	Work on sense of touch first by touching the skin (with light, medium and deep pressure) on arms, legs and torso and hold touch points.	Clear stress of touch using Gv16, Bl9 and Bl62. If touch is still stressful try Pc6.
Focus and Concentration	Listening to sound exercise and for concentration try the drive and determination points	Bl52 – drive and determination

Memory	Listening to sound exercise and the points related to opening up to your heart	Pc6 – opening up to your heart
Writing	Improve coordination and balance first then write and hold points	Bl9 and Bl10
Speech	Improve coordination and balance first then work with speech.	Speech – Gv15 and GB20
Stroke	Balance	Bl10 and Bl9
	Marching homolateral & cross lateral	Bl62 and Gv16
	Emotional Stress	Bl9
Able to plan and implement tasks to meet deadlines, understanding time	Try improving coordination and balance in order to develop logic function	Same sided marching – Gv16 and Bl9; opposite side Bl62 (can also try Gv16 and Bl9) Balance – Bl9, Bl10
Catching	Improve same sided marching first then opposite side marching, balance and vision	Same sided marching – Gv16 and Bl9; opposite side Bl62 (can also try Gv16 and Bl9) Balance – Bl9, Bl10 Vision St1 and GB20
Disturbed sleep	Close eyes and imagine sleeping	Bl62

Confused thinking	Improve same sided marching first then opposite side marching, balance and then use the clarity of thinking points	Same sided marching – Gv16 and Bl9; opposite side Bl62 (can also try Gv16 and Bl9) Balance – Bl9, Bl10 Clarity of thinking GB20
Emotional stress and anxiety	Think of the stress and anxiety and hold points	Bl9, Gv16 and Bl62
Depression	Think of the depression and hold points	Pc6
Stressed about the future or past	Visualise future or past event while you hold points	Bl62 or Gv16
Autism	Work on sense of touch first by touching the skin (with light, medium and deep pressure) on arms, legs and torso and hold touch points. Improve marching and balance first, then focus on hearing and vision.	Clear stress of touch using Gv16, Bl9 and Bl62. If touch is still stressful try Pc6. Same sided marching Gv16 and Bl9; Opposite side Bl62 (can also try Gv16 and Bl9) Balance – Bl9, Bl10
Attention Deficit syndrome	Apply power tools in the order of the book. Particularly focus on marching, balance, hearing, vision (see above), and touch (see above). Then try focus and concentration.	Same sided marching Gv16 and Bl9; Opposite side Bl62 (can also try Gv16 and Bl9) Balance – Bl9, Bl10 Vision, hearing, touch, focus and concentration – see above
Cerebellum disorders	March and balance holding points	Bl9, Bl10, Gv16

CONCLUSION

The techniques in this book can make a large difference to how well your brain functions in life. We have made use of ancient wisdom and applied it to modern problems using acupressure and movement.

My vision is to use this work to help empower people to make the most of their lives. These techniques have made a major difference to thousands of people worldwide. If you feel inspired to learn more I encourage you to find out more about Kinesiology or Holistic Kinesiology or on Brain Function courses from the following websites – from Germany www.iak-.fe and from Australia www.complementary.com.au